COVID THRU EYES OF ESSENTIAL WORKER

Pandemic is really Life

Reid Skillset

ISBN: 978-1-915147-62-2 (PAPERBACK)

Book Design by Aeyshaa

CONTENTS

Somewhere during the coronavirus pandemic! As the death toll grew inexplicably to 1.28 million worldwide deaths! And a growing number of people are affected by the virus daily. Exactly 51.9 million, during the time of writing. It became very clear or downright obvious. How the virus was desensitized by world leaders. Especially a home of a brave president!

There become all types of myths and hypotheticals. Besides wearing masks to the cleanliness of hands, with either soap or sanitizer to social distancing. Also a warmer weather concept or theory. That maintains the virus. This is why I decided to write a book on the infodemic. I will give all information. I can be based on coronavirus from a first-hand experience!

This book I am writing is not a mock shift. As I researched a lot of this thoroughly and looked into mitigating factors to date. I in no way or any way possible. Will never make a mockery of this very deadly virus. I only wanted to give proficient information to help cope with the loss and other aspects. May it be from coronavirus aka covid-19, it's vaccinations or booster shots!

Whether it be helping you find your sanity during the highest times of debt and depression. Since the Great Depression! Or give a scenario in which vaccinations conquer covid-19! Also the very possible side effects of a vaccine. And its threat to the people.

#1 ESSENTIAL

A big reason why I decided to write this book about coronavirus and its vaccinations. Is because I was oblivious to the deadly virus. I can remember a homeboy about a month before the pandemic hit telling friends to prepare for a recession. What I would see in a matter of months. After his proclamation. Would be very disheartening!

The deadly coronavirus would morph in a matter of weeks. Due to inefficient or lack of respect for people (death toll)! And the validity of effects of coronavirus worldwide! Firsthand I worked as an essential worker. In a grocery store.

I mean I remember hearing rumors of lockdown. Well for me the hearsay would turn full-throttle. When I received a letter from the front office of my job about travel commute to and from work during a lockdown! I knew then my life was about to change upside down! How much? Of course not!

The date was around the end of February 2020. The talk of the town had caused mayhem in the grocery store. People for some odd reason began to stockpile or better word-hoard. Everything from food to toiletries to hand sanitizer to disinfectants. I can remember vividly posting on social media. "America wasn't built for mass hysteria!"

There hadn't been a declared pandemic. Yet people were already acting like idiots. A better word would be savages! I can remember an incident where I and another co-worker physically helped an older defenseless family. That was de-moralizing. Those days at work I will admit. I was dejected. There is, being a spiritually enlightened person! I prayed for people in silence!

Unbeknownst to me. At the time we would need more prayers from world leaders. Also diligent efforts to lockdown areas. The lack of negligence would soon be sprawled all over America and the world.

#2
QUARANTINE

The official day was March 11, 2020. The coronavirus aka covid_19 had gained control over almost all of the world. People would be confined to homes. Unless deemed essential. See at the exact time, I wouldn't notice being termed essential.

Probably was way too much for me mentally. All I knew then was if you came in contact with a person who had contracted cornonavirus aka covid-19. You had to quarantine for 14 days. There was a list of things that were deemed essential. From your local gas station to bodegas, to pharmacies, and last but not least grocery stores.

I mean never in times did it seem to be a dangerous unhealthy or toxic place to be at work. But soon to be the heightened scare had everybody affected. People became upset in grocery stores getting into fights in aisle 12. Over any household thing, you could name. From steaks to sanitizer that sold out.

The fortunes weren't looking good. The things that were usually in stock. It wasn't on shelves. People became confused. People became impatient! With that came frustration.

We were now in a bind working. A real bad working space. I can remember the look from a customer staring at and looking for an invisible piece of steak to appear. Then the infamous, "Hey buddy you out of steak?" It was clear it didn't take a rocket scientist to tell you were looking at an empty rack. *I knew my people were about to be served up a real entre!*

While working, I tried to keep a good positive mind frame. But to see bustling cities have no signs of human movement was demoralizing! Their businesses began to flounder. People fell on hard times!

The deadly coronavirus had wreaked havoc on precious land. It felt like a black plague had fallen on places of color. In my local area, people had to become really resourceful and remain safe.

In other cluster cities. Where the high population in the dense inner city. Almost made it impossible to really social distance. The numbers grew even higher. It became what it seemed like it was! A death sentence for elderly people of color!

If you are like me you began to question! While others began to lose hope fighting for the last whatever. We began to go into a cruel time. People didn't care about the elderly.

Nursing homes were locked as hospitalizations soared out of control. Never at any time of my life, from the people. I asked had we seen something. Matter of fact, anything like this?

#3
LOCKDOWN

To think that in 2020 people would be confined to their homes isn't beyond unimaginable. But the measures were needed earlier. If you look at the true meaning of lockdown.

It has a lot to do with confining and isolating as a security measure to regain control. Basically saying, people were stripped of some of their freedom! The outbreak was serious and protective measures were needed.

Especially in these cluster cities, the coronavirus was never maintained from the start. So the most drastic moves were made. The public was remanned to stay-at-home procedure. There was a public health crisis. If there was a glimmer of hope. It was slim.

The lockdown was not only devasting to independent people. But also nonessential businesses such as other retail stores, gyms, barbershops, and salons.

At no time had people encured this in the modern-day era. Home of the free! This crushed the totality of the demographic of the economy! And worst mental health, and family structure!

Quarantining became the norm unless you were a frontline worker or essential worker. I just happened to fall in later. Creativity and high-level resourcefulness became a priority. People had to do a lot of soul-searching.

During the highest time of positivity rates from coronavirus (covid-19) infections. Listening to the persuasive or abrasive orders came with people. Not being as disciplined to orders as freedom always shows.

Climate change had a major part in this. With the warm weather emerging during the pandemic. That warm weather was accepted. By most conspiracy theorists.

Soon people would be flocking to parks. Needing to escape the isolation of their living quarters. Next, they were pictures of packed beaches. It became clear that people didn't react well to direct orders!

The sanity of people or remaining sane was no doubt tested! By the public crisis of coronavirus (covid-19) during the pandemic. When I say tested? I should write tempted!

Meaning there were all types of temptations to escape or evade the isolation. As well as a little added incentive to drink alcohol because liquor stores. Just happened to be also deemed essential.

The Lockdown left people feeling desolate. Let me break it down. People had a desire to do something. Whether wrong or right. Even if it meant being a determent to your health or others with possible coronavirus infection.

It was blatant that people didn't like or accept being away from other people. Or being treated like prisoners in their own homes.

As safe as our government officials told us our homes would be. That solitary confinement began to break the interior and exterior of people. This can happen to the most ruthless of people.

Or to the most subtle or humble. We never would understand! The total effect this lockdown would have on alcoholism and mental health. From depression to anxiety to p.t.s.d. Calculations from this pandemic soared.

Millions of people fell on hard times financially. Which caused a trickle-down effect mentally and physically! There become all types of questions about mental health, anxiety, depression, alcoholism, and last but not least domestic violence. There was no doubt people were struggling with day-to-day activities.

The toll of being financially unstable and insecure from being unemployed. Destroyed souls and spirits. To go along with the country deeming liquor stores essential. That was mixology 101 at its best. We were encouraging a new problem for some. That we hadn't experienced. Since the prohibition era!

The sad reality is America birthed some undisciplined rebellious alcoholics at the wrong damn time. I mean the types who never struggled with alcohol because maybe their age didn't co-exist with the pandemic. But there's always a method to the madness.

#4
FLATTEN THE CURVE

As coronavirus ran rampant. I can remember starting to see some people wear those big biological warfare masks! Also, other P.P.E masks. Known as Full-face, Half-face masks, and N-95. These are all Protective Personal Equipment.

While wearing the first mask compared to last was a little overboard. I thought at the time. But who am I to tell someone. "How to protect themselves and families"

As I look back on those days. I have to admit chemical warfare was thought of by many conspiracy theorists! From onset. So if wearing protection. From pathogens was viable means of adding longevity to your life, family, and others. That's what you do.

You don't run to packed parks and beaches. For the added risk of exposure. Just for some cheap thrills! We would need safety measures, guidelines, and solutions from the Government! State officials or other leaders to "Deflate." The number of coronavirus (covid-19) infections and deaths!

On April 15, 2020. New mandates were made to slow the spread of coronavirus. All people were to wear facial masks in public. This meant people were to wear masks in groceries, pharmacies, gas stations, and other essential businesses.

The measure was very much needed in cluster cities. From the beginning. In areas where another mandate might be impossible to achieve. Social distancing was termed by leaders.

As much as you bring in the coast guard to help facilitate physical distancing. There's nothing you can do. When people live on top of each other like in inner cities.

In means the trajectory was great. Trying to socially distance yourself isn't impossible. But in densely populated cluster cities. Remaining six feet apart or two-arm lengths out. Became a task all in itself.

Running regular errands was a challenge. People were panicky in stores. Obvious note with the yelling. "Get Back!" To the most harmless or unintimidating person wearing a mask. Who just happened to invade their social distancing space.

There became instructions. Directions for patrons with little footsteps and arrows to help guide people! Especially the shoppers to maintain social distancing.

By this time trepidation had set in. People were fearful of coronavirus (covid-19) infections or deaths. There was a need for a definite solution. Another step in curving the virus was washing hands thoroughly for 30 seconds with soap and water or hand sanitizer. The cleanliness of washing hands. I thought was self-explanatory. But the price gauging of hand sanitizer became horrendous and intolerable.

The hoarding of any disinfectant sprays, wipes, and alcohol products made them scarce. It was impossible to keep them on shelves. Anywhere because of the high public demand. For those specific items without supply. That again put a dark cloud over the people. If coronavirus aka (covid-19) hadn't plagued us enough already.

Flattening the curve of coronavirus wasn't going to be any simple task. It was going to take neccessary steps. As high positivity rates were at the forefront. Death was right in front of your face. People were losing loved ones.

I can remember a school friend! He was one of the first that I can say. I knew to go. This was a guy who I played high school football with me. A happy spirited and physically fit. Just gone!

As much as we questioned health standards and protocols. We the people would have to follow the guidelines and directions. If we wanted to conquer this pandemic.

It's not like the instructions were extremely hard to follow. A lot I feel was self-explanatory! Especially when looking at it like. They are life or death consequences and complications. I mean underlying health factors or issues. Meaning the elderly and older people who had previous health implications.

Whether it be from asthma to lung disease to heart disease to cancer. Coronavirus was taking people out at a faster rate. There was really only one who could save us from covid-19. And when a state leader pronounced, "God will not save us from covid-19!" I knew we were in big trouble.

A death sentence was ordered for people all around the world. While people still proceeded to move mercifully around. Galavanting at the family card game. Unknowingly risking family members' lives!

Not seeing the mistake. In their lapse of judgment. Own family members were at fault for the deaths! As much as we blame hospitals. For negligence or miscalculations. However you look at it, you have to look at it with clarity! To make sure? We blame people for the same exact lack of accountability also.

Now if you are a kid. We understand. But any adult. Especially elderly adults in hands of family health care. This news was extremely devasting. I mean people knew of the risk of exposure. We just didn't know how deadly coronavirus's effects on the world would be. It's the worst plague known to mankind in this present day.

Inconspicuous to most there was only one who could flatten the curve. And he wasn't giving any orders, instructions, or directions. As plagues have been around since the beginning of time. From the Spanish flu pandemic at the start of February 1918. Which had over 50,000,000 deaths.

Also 500 million suspected cases. As much as we know that no specific medicine stopped or ended that epidemic. All we know is a resilient spiritual people dealt with lots of loss!

Oh and 102 years later that Spain was not where the pandemic originated. But where, it was first reported by the news. Is beyond mystifying!

As coronavirus moved along leaving a catastrophic effect on society's health. It also left a grappling hardship on people's finances. Not only were people getting sick and dying from covid! The economy due to lockdown started to fall into a recession. With nonessential businesses closed. Families struggled and started to run through savings. Most weren't working because of closings.

Soon millions would be filling out unemployment insurance applications online trying to make means and provide for families. The more time passed began rumors of relief payout to families! Which was needed as some people had entered dire straits and ruts.

Struggling to pull themselves out. I could only imagine how hard. It was literally! For the average families living below the median across the country.

With words of rumors began speculation. Of payouts from the government. Everything from a hero's package for frontline and essential workers! To economic relief for struggling families. There were no means. Most by now had lost everything from businesses to everyday social life.

A new birth was being formed or should I say a re-birth. Some of our old ways were being compromised. Not only physically. But of course financially! I always say a line a fucked up person isn't going to rationalize well. If you think that out. You will see the perspective. I mean the amounts they were saying for some were outrageous. But the latter was needed for now non-working families.

On March 27, 2020, our elected president. Then signed a historic 2 trillion dollar stimulus package! To help the American public and US economy reeling from covid-19. That day as we knew things changed forever. It was no more of the old and original! But a more of out with old in with new!

If you look at the meaning of new. It means to not exist before, be made, introduced, or discovered recently or now for the first time. Then normal which means conforming to a standard, usual, typical, or expected. That combined should have warned some of us. Even prepared some of us. For the unexpected changing of the guard!

I mean nowhere in time. As I can remember did people have the time to personally isolate themselves? Really find that creative space to notice what they were personally passionate about! Motivated about I mean as much as the world needed payouts for struggling families. No amount of money could fix what some lost.

The numbers just didn't add up. But what did was. We needed to be able to combine our creative natures and get in touch with our inner selves and beings. There adapting to advanced technological measures. We moved toward. A soon too be, new revolutionalized world.

While I was still going to work as an essential worker. At the grocery store. Children were attending schools on tele-conferences. Which showed the efficiency and effectiveness of a new platform. Results were everywhere. Stocks for that specific brand soared through the roof.

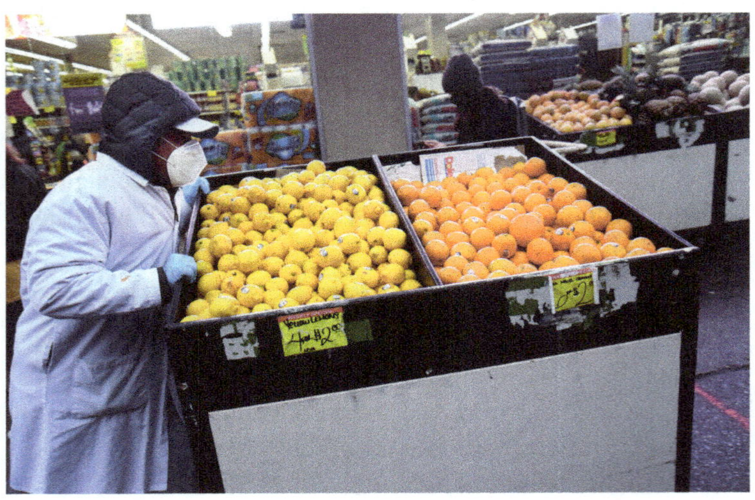

Things were slowly changing. People were showing resiliency. At the store, I tried to understand as much as cutting back hours was now hurting me. I still had a gig. I managed my everyday life and tried to become efficient in my own specific way.

#6
RESOURCEFUL

From the standard point of writing this book. I have to admit pre covid! People who shopped at the store. Were a little more courteous. And as much as a co-workers said "entitled." I have to admit. She was right. I mean no where in the common world did coming off rude get you anywhere.

But in the pandemic people had lost their morals. Better yet marbles. It's like people didn't appreciate the isolated feeling. Or the disservice of going without. That same feeling developed in some of our inner beings. The ability to be creative in an empty space.

At other times, the job was starting to get on my nerves. I got into with customers who were full of games. I personally asked to be a freezer box. So I didn't have to deal with the customers. I thought that was reasonable. Since I had run out of patience. Also since the store was starting to runoff incompetence, dysfunction, and mayhem.

It was like a mad house in there. The pace of shoppers was very different. Most didn't adapt well to having to find clever ways to overcome difficulties. Besides with speed!

That adrenaline rush combined with a panic attack formed a very toxic workspace. As much as I tried to distance myself.

There was nothing I could do. The lack of common courtesy and overall unresourcefulness was getting to everybody. People were impatient and confused.

See most of the stuff we kept on shelves was impossible to import because of stopped shipping from country to country. That meant some of the store's most valuable commodities.

Or the hot seller at the store was out of stock! That destroyed the demographic of some people who weren't resourceful enough. I give you a prime example of how it happened.

One day as a restaurant owner looked at me with a baffled look. He asked, "Hey Buddy! When you think you getting fresh salmon?" I answered. " Where have you been? We been out of fresh salmon about a month?" He was shocked. But aware of the answer in the statement.

This guy was a regular. So I felt his struggle. I referred the next best option! Which was frozen salmon. He answered exact words. "That's shit!" I shrugged my shoulders and lifted my two arms to the side. Then responded. "You're going to have to be resourceful!" Then preceded to do the rest of my work.

As life played its way out like it always does. About a week and a half later. As I rushed into work one day. I saw a familiar face in the frozen seafood area. Loading boxes of frozen salmon onto a cart. I couldn't help but laugh. Then as I sneakingly unknowingly got closer to him. I said exact words, " I thought that was shit?" He laughed and replied, "RE-SOURCEFUL." I responded, "VERY RESOURCEFUL!"

#7
RUMORS AND SKEPTICISM

While hospitalizations contineud to soar from corona-virus covid-19. The most disheartening thing was the closings of nursing homes. Now I understand this was mandatory protocol for flattening the curve of coronavirus. I am like most of the world.

I just didn't know the impact of those pictures. Of loved ones touching window-glass! Reciprocating love would have on somebody's mental health status then. Even now! Also the treatment of older people. While being served unexplainably a death sentence! Shcok the cores of families.

During these times, there began talks or rumors of innovative medicines. That would reduce the effectiveness of coronavirus. A cocktail shct! That began with infamous medical procedures. Had public in an uprise because of conspiracy theorists' take on being lab rats.

It made people question the authoritative measures. The misinformation was so indirect. It felt like something was top secret while people died. Experimental testing was at the forefront.

People at the job talked or cooked up the notion or theory of taking an immunization shot. That freed you of coronavirus aka (covid-19). From the customers to the workers there was a mutual dissatisfaction with the thought.

See looking back at the time. I can see why so many were imposed to it. From the beginning. Nobody wanted to look like the test dummy. But as numbers continued to soar. The worry or desperation for answers would contribute to our soon quality of life!

The skepticism of a vaccine should have been expected. Things were looking slimmer by the day. I was working consistently. But I started to second guess. And question?

Was all the maneuvering around from desolate city to city worth it. Well financially at the time. I thought I was. It wasn't like I was doing any better. I just thought. I was being self-sufficient as I could be. Boy was I wrong!

See at the time. As I worked in that hectic crafty maneuvering work environment. I wasn't in the best mental space. I mean I consider myself. A great guy during the time.

But something was going on under the surface. Who gets all the right insight at the right time. I would directly have to walk some moves out to find out. Literally! What really was going on?

#8
ORANGE ZONE

Sometimes we never understand colors. Or how they correlate to what we are going through on a day-to-day basis. I worked at the store for over a year now.

Honestly I felt confident because of my work ethic. I really appreciated having a job. Something about working during that time at moments. Did feel like? It was giving me extra incentives to go to work.

My commute was usually a now super quiet empty bus ride. Throughout the process. There was more excruciating stuff on me. Then I had ever prepared myself for mentally.

Looking back working in that job. At times, changed my life forver. My thought process was to go to work! Get a check. Save and do all again. But one of the days. As I was walking to work. After exiting the bus ride. I started to notice long lines at local health clinics.

The first day it was seemingly odd. That I observed it because it was minimal for what was going on. A lot of it was expected because people were planning. To now travel because of the upcoming holiday season. Had me especially sort of on the edge at the store.

The next day. As I approached the same area where I noticed the line the first time. This time. It was significantly longer! From the eye, something wasn't right. I mean I thought all the process of flattening the curve was working. I guess I was being optimistic, hopeful, and downright naive.

By then, I had asked some co-workers about? The conditions in the surrounding neighborhood and at the store. I was surprised to find out from a co-worker. Not front office! That the city. We worked in had just morphed from a yellow zone to an orange zone. Meaning that the area had elevated positivity rates from coronavirus aka covid-19.

Once I heard that I began to panic. Just like a hypochondriac! See not only was coronavirus working on me mentally. That day at the job.

Honestly, I felt like it had the upper hand on me. I remember feeling visibly shaken. I know didn't give that off. But under the surface, I was perspiring harder. Then I ever sweated at work.

The next few days at the job. I was extremely uneasy. Especially since those lines. I saw got longer and longer. I decided to go speak with the front office and union representative. Just trying to make sure safety measures were made in an attempted effort to protect us! The workers.

For the number of people touching stuff . It just didn't make sense. Trying to make sure they were sanitizing everything in the store. Mainly I did that by making sure the company was following mandates. Protecting us as the area was infected.

Now I can look back and understand everything. See with the changing of hue. It brought positive and negative interactions. Just like coronavirus had done from start.

We can correlate it with seasons. How we feel better in nicer spring and summer. And a little bit more bummer for winter and fall. What confused me? Then and now is an epiphany all itself. The color orange during covid was associated with death!

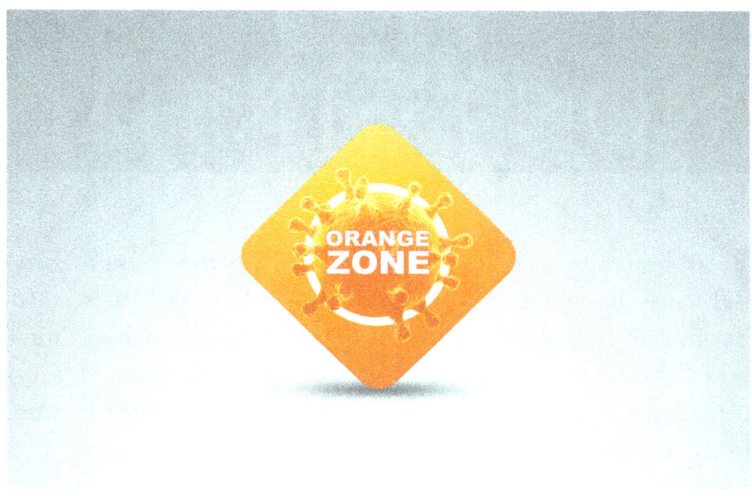

But in reality, the true meaning of orange on a real color scale means Joy and creativity! It's very clear coronavirus had us confused.

Looking back at those exact days during the orange zone. I'm noticing I was really observant! I think I was starting to pay attention to minor details. Especially when didn't co-exist with a mandated protocol for coronavirus. It's no top secret anymore now. That I can admit like almost everbody. I was scared to death of that shit!

Literally, I watched to see how much the store took into account. What I said to them in the front office. Not following safety rules for a business could lead to major setbacks. But since I had already watched the store turn into a madhouse.

I circled back and spoke with the union rep. Who just happened to be making the same point of the heightened scare of coronavirus and orange zone! In the surrounding area. And of course at the store. "They needed to have more people wiping down and sanitizing areas."

Now as this went on. I couldn't help but be wearier and more leary of people in leadership. I know the representation was able to get information to them.

I also watched the interaction of the sanitizing guy. Which was one guy a shift. Who maintained grounds! That was mainly carts and trash. But over a few days. I noticed the job had put more on their specific workload.

So sanitizing came with a little added extra incentive. What I didn't know was. How they neglected and negotiated some of their own incompetence.

Especially at the top! See I know you can't wipe an area every single second. As much as I wanted. That were the precautionary steps the mandate had set! What I do know is they could have controlled the risks. By not letting as many people in at times. Now I understand that some of these people were business owners. What I didn't understand?

Is how some bigger businesses thrived off the dysfunction. Which caters to customers. But also risks their workers! While the smaller business. That who worked hard and lived by the mandate were crushed. Those who lived under those same business standards. But the business failed miserably. I guess showed me that "Business is business!"

Visible seeing that messed with my head. I remember a young beautiful lady. Who had her nice little cafe right in the middle of the vibrant section of her town!

Had to make her feel like. She made it. But again she lived by the protocol. And possibly fell victim to covid herself and itself. I noticed when I didn't see her for a while.

She was a regular and got the same thing almost every time. While always keeping a good mind frame. I questioned why more customers weren't like her.

When I did finally see her online. The protocol was serving a purpose. But serving to the inspector's eye only. Somewhere I guess. To know and see this woman's business go under. Wasn't the most ideal situation for us at the job.

We all needed to see somebody like us. Help us to keep our day going. She was that for me! I worked hard some days.

But my energy didn't match. I started to look at it like I was taking a 45-minute commute from a safe zone. Into a hot zone. Which now the orange comparatively maintained and represented.

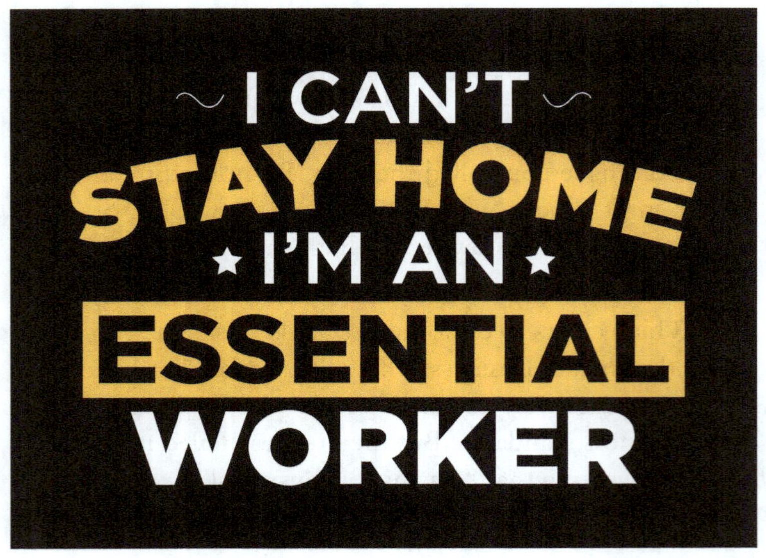

Barber shops, hair salons, and all other non-essential businesses were still closed. I concluded! It was my time to go. The hours didn't add up. I was making pennies.

I mean, not only was I not making enough. Now just the thought! Of catching coronavirus and maybe dying or bringing it back to my family. That scenario played out. All over and over again. So much it startled me. I left working as an essential worker.

#10
CREATIVE DESIGN AND DIRECTION

See working in retail. During covid was no doubt a blessing in disguise. I always remained grateful for being gainfully employed. I came home from prison, maybe a year prior. So working hard and putting blinders on was nothing new to me.

But what I dealt with customers became outright disrespectful. To think I almost came to blows with customers. Is beyond ridiculous! But hey it's like a co-worker said entitlement. I remember pre-covid.

The store was so gentle and quiet. Those days. She was roaring loud and steaming hot. Filled with customers with built-up financially repressed aggressiveness.

I think I'm a social guy. I feel I can almost get along with anybody. As long as you don't disrespect my intelligence. Or unless we clash on moral principle issues.

I will say this. I nor any of my co-workers were ever in any wrong. When supply and demand were through the roof. I know I tried to maintain a great perspective throughout working during covid in a grocery store.

But it became clear just because you spending money! *It doesn't make the customer right. Especially when the customer has no service.*

That same entitlement made me leave my job. The insecurities of plague and or sickness. Had clouded my overall thinking. See I walked away from my job. Living my little self-sufficient life. Never noticing I had did something?

What I forgot was I didn't have a job. I didn't have any means at all. As I tried to figure out. What was going on with covid? I pieced my life back together.

Sustainability is a big word. Just like sufficiency is. See at the time. I was working hard. But not for financial freedom. I mean I was still financially illiterate.

I had no clue about generating enough creativity. That could start a small business. Even if I was sitting on one! It would take some time for things to play out.

Leaving the store at that exact time. It wasn't the best timing. As the holiday season was very soon approaching. There already was a backup with unemployment. That had been for months. Already stifling people. I can personally say coronavirus was crippling people.

I didn't know where my next check was going to come from. But I stayed positive throughout. Somewhere deep down. I knew I had just decided to protect my family from covid! Also my mental health space. A big step in creative growth.

In a matter of weeks. I felt the decision financially. I started to stress out. I knew the odds of getting unemployment because I quit were slim. I still was going to apply.

At that time, as I started to look around for work. I came up with an idea for a book about coronavirus aka covid-19. Since I just worked in a grocery store as an essential worker. I was ecstatic about the idea. All I could think of was. "It can't get any more creative than that."

I could remember vividly. As the holiday season grew closer and closer. Friends and families started to question my motives. I guess gauging where I was at? Emotionally, physically, and last but not least financially.

See for me. I sort of knew! I was going to take a hit financially. I knew I was going to have to sacrifice. Did I know at the time? How much? No question. NOT!!!

I started to outline. As much as I could from scenarios of events and a timeline with coronavirus. I then started to journal, record, and screenshot. Everything I got about coronavirus.

The more I delved deep into the research. I became amazed at scientific facts. Not just hypotheticals or scenarios. Data-driven information. That can correct errors and pivot into creative ideas with technology and design.

Getting into the writing for me was fun. Self relenting. It felt like I was now destined for writing. There was happiness in me from creative expression!

That makes me think and made me a little sad. That it really took coronavirus aka covid-19 deaths. And protecting my mental health and family to notice my imagination of original ideas.

As we finished up one holiday. In grand fashion with still high positivity rates! From coronavirus via holiday travel. I felt I was blessed to be in a free creative space. Which I was but again. I had no clue!

The fear of the unknown had everybody tripping and bugging out. At that same time! As word of more testing for now coronavirus vaccinations went on.

I think the closer we got to those trial dates and rumors of such. It just didn't sit well with people who wanted freedom. Not isolation. The fear of an unknown shot. Only intensified people's behaviors.

Arguments occurred over the smallest of stuff. People were becoming more judgmental by the day. Shit second, minute, and hour. Whatever you prefer. Time was of the essence!

This was widespread. People weren't there as much as they claimed emotionally, physically, and financially like they said they were. People were just downright trying to be evil and crush dreams.

I'm giving you. An example, as time passed. We got closer to the season of holiday giving. My close friends thought it was cool. To pull us up on some real things. That night a lot of my life was critiqued.

I didn't know from going. Into that, they felt I was being a crutch or they were enabling me with help. They spoke about it earlier. I was confused. I took everything with a grain of salt though.

Especially when the idea of me doing a book about covid-19 came up. Laughter erupted. It's like I was being ridiculed for trying to do something.

I thought was informative, influential, and helpful. I just listened and agreed to look for work. But when I heard somebody say the exact words "Scrap that book!" I will admit that was when I felt covid had defeated me.

I went through those holidays at my lowest point. I was down in out. For a few weeks. I had problems fathoming what was happening. Right as the holiday came and went! Numbers rose. Dramatically where schools had to be closed again! Drew a rise from everybody. For me, that was a blessing in disguise. I needed that empty space. Too find elation in creation.

I stayed to myself and one day. As I cleaned up. I looked at the book I started to write. Then I had thought to throw it out. But something wouldn't let me. Let go of it. I held it for about 2 or 3 minutes. Contemplating getting rid of the book or not?

Something just didn't sit right with me. I could remember vividly thinking of this as great informative information. That can help vaccinations, immunizations, and possible side effects.

I felt this work had a place in history that nobody could speak of. The authentication at time. Literally and honestly didn't just go with the book. I honestly felt passionate about not throwing it out!

So I didn't. I just put the book down and recalibrated my thoughts. On finances. I knew times were hard for a lot of people. From the growing number of new positive coronavirus infections from holiday travel. To unemployment and job closures.

The economy for most families was bleak. I embraced looking for work. But with sicknesses getting worse. Finding gainful employment was a task in itself. I immediately second-guessed myself.

#12 OPERATION WARP SPEED

The medical procedure of vaccinations for coronavirus was expedited extremely fast. The test trial runs were so top secret. That nobody knew of the true effectiveness and efficiency of the vaccine. Or the side effects.

All we knew was. The numbers of deaths were so high. That a scare tactic remained! A conspiracy theorist's dream of thinking. It was in no way possible. It was created. Then clinically tested. In the amount of emergency timing. Maybe I'm a conspiracist too. I guess? Or more of an educated realist.

To hear about any medicine mentioned with warp and speed. Especially one that was destined to slow sickness of coronavirus. Which killed at a wickedly rapid pace. By numbers, coronavirus had killed more people than lung disease, heart disease, and cancer. And at a faster rate. Then any other plague in any modern history.

Once you were hooked to a ventilator many didn't make it back off. There were even shortages of ventilators. Equipment was maneuvered around with limited success because of high positivity rates across the country.

Emergency rooms were converted to makeshifts. Negative air. Which was needed for decontamination! Was extremely overwhelming for nurses, doctors, and families of covid victims.

I mean you can't expect a delibated people to accept an unheard-of medicine. The more we found out. It was a shot and some other form of immunization. Some people totally rejected the idea. Including myself!

I get it looking back. Nobody wanted to be a guinea pig. To be tested, poked, and prodded. With God knows whatever in needles. Last but not least truth be told.

That maybe it was us preventing or alleviating us from covid-19. Crept people the fuck out. I mean in no time did we trust the health system. But the misinformation was very evident as a friend had told me. Whose family worked in a hospital since covid emerged. There were only 4 flu deaths.

There had to be miscalculations somewhere. Something didn't add up? Also, a stealth new sleek medicine bomber was on its way!

One of the meanings of warp is to contort or bend out of shape. Now as we look, at speed. It has a lot to do with the rate or at which someone or something can operate something!

Last but not least. Organization. Which is simplifying organizing something. If you combine altogether the different phrases. You get the full contextual meaning of what was going on.

Deception has long been a tool to trick and confuse people into doing things. Since the beginning of time.

We always fall for the ole 52 fake-out. As much as now I know. What I'm writing about looking back! Again I didn't know what was going on at time. And who to believe. It definitely wasn't going to be from some media circuit.

While most news media had daily coverage of the progress of this new change in the world of medicine. The trial processes were real tight-lipped as you would expect from a country.

That showed the deceit and misinformation. I was so highly opposed to vaccines from the start. There wasn't a person on earth. I believed could of changed that! Well, it would be. It just had nothing to do with excessive speed.

#13
JOURNALING

At the same time as I became enamored with daily theatrics with coronavirus aka covid-19! I had an idea. I would record, jot, and word in the best possible day-to-day format! I think when I had the thought. It was the presence of the unknown creative therapy.

The exact moment in time. I had no inclination. How maybe that personal suggestion to a course of action! Would start to lead me to one of my ultimate dilemmas.

I started this journaling. In the beginning of the tenth month of year 2020! Coronavirus was still wreaking havoc and our medical stealth mission. Had become center stage.

The effects were felt as people continued to die at a high rate. The first day of collecting some of the information wasn't anything special. I felt at the time. It had no meaning. I had to learn to record your work, Is a thing of greatness!

We question ourselves. But when questioned with death! We humans, go crazy. It's like some of us. Don't know how to accept the principle of death! You have to live to die.

I think starting to journal those first few days. My directed creative energy was as early as a red-eye! I took to it. I was amazed by some of the statisical stats. But remember at the time. I respected everything.

I was also very suspicious! To any new methods. Mainly because like most. We had never heard of or personally been through a plague like this.

I think one thing that led to the research. Breaking down the sciences of what they were saying daily. Wasn't at all about any state leaders' slogans, mottos, and gimmicks.

People were dying. Especially the elderly. The numbers as they grew became scary. I enjoyed hearing the little information. I got. I didn't know. But I sort of knew.

If I did diligent work on coronavirus, vaccines, and side-effects. I felt comfortable on my side. Of not ever taking it!

Each day at the top of the morning! I watched almost each and every news media circuit! Trying to gain as much insight. Some of the information was repetitive. But I tried to see.

As much as possible on coronavirus and its vaccinations. I didn't want to miss anything! There would be no pulling the wool over these eyes.

Before this time. Journaling was never a hobby of mine. I will admit. I enjoyed writing. Just didn't fully understand the daily therapeutic creative side of journaling! I felt the need to do the work because there was an epidemic and a public health scare.

But without the emergence of coronavirus aka covid-19. I sort of wonder? If I would have found this stuff out!

The day-to-day writing made me eager to find out more. See I had extra incentive because I took life seriously. So, as I researched all aspects of coronavirus and vaccinations. There was a hunger for more types of information, cause, and effect. That I would need to nourish. Like my life and family's lives depended on it.

#14 HOLIDAY TRAVEL SPIKE

With the Holiday season in primed season. Or right around the corner. Are esteemed colleagues of Rhode scholars and doctors. Predicted or estimated that these times would be more vicious.

They also advised most to stay home and live by standard set. With inefficiency or inability to sit still. Really incompetency. Most Americans started to plan to visit family or attend anytime getaway.

The Head of doctor at the infectious disease center predicted this all with maybe some intel. That shit scares the shit out of me to think anyway otherwise.

Anyways I was spooked at those exact moments. I was still following protocol. And looked at some theorists as covid-iddiots. Meaning they knew so much as far in terms of family. But was still able, willing, and ready to go somewhere! Knowing you had the chance of getting sick. Also then possiblity to bring it back to the family. Added to the death toll!

I remember seeing these images of bodies loaded up in trucks. Truckloads of bodies. It was like the death rate.

Covid-19 was leaving was faster. Then previous regimes of death had left. And the amounts of cemeteries they had just could not hold. The amount of death!

I don't think any country was prepared for this. We were all blindsided by coronavirus. Of course, a lot of curving covid-19! Was going to take paying attention. To the new strict medical orders and procedures. The type where the public! Actually listens and follows orders. Was a total different story though!

Maybe I was disciplined or designed to mentally wither through the storm of covid. But will I admit? I was blatantly shitless scared of covid! Yessir or ma'am. I can remember at those times being visibly shaken.

Those images and the rising rate of death. Coupled together added more confusion. To the why? I mean nobody wanted to die. From some new virus.

So I stayed to myself. I started to try to be seen less. Keeping a real discreet demeanor. As far as amounts of people I was around. The risk was growing each day from exposure to positive people. The logic didn't make sense for me to go to South Beach during the holiday season!

But for some it did! There were a lot of incompetent ideas during covid-19 from the public. I can understand the uproar from potential possible vaccinations. What I didn't understand? Was for people to travel to hot zone cities and states. Then think they would be no stipulations! When returning home was beyond stupid and redundant.

Ok, I get it. The travel was more feasible. People were able to visit places at lower prices because of the impact covid-19 left on econmy. Many jumped at the opportunity! While many will blame holiday travel for this coronavirus holiday spike.

But honestly, it was more than that. Just like in one of America's greatest grandest sports. When it came to cheap travel. Combined with rebellious citizens who could get others sick including family. Many balked at that opportunity.

The high risk of death. Is what really spooked me. Like was this really a death sentence for elderly and older senior citizens. The treatment they received was horrendous. And people moved along without a care. A lot being anti-this. The theory remained people were going to travel. Wherever, Whenever, and However! But at whose expense?

I remember losing my Uncle to covid during this time. So it stung! This was my Dad's brother. Like some of the last of a dying breed of male lineage! That I knew from the past.

So the effect was a little different. I felt the pain when I spoke to my family. The hurt of deception. A cover-up! All I knew was. I wasn't going down to the funeral! As it was advised for me not to go. See some people can get the message before it's sent.

Coronavirus wrecked more havoc. Then any other pandemic or plague in modern history. And to think it was played with and downplayed by leaders and the public. Is a downright travesty.

I mean in no time in present history as we know. Did people not only not follow. But actually, couldn't sit their asses down. For sake of family, friends, and others.

Was perceived very well by people in high authority. But beyond unimaginable for the public. There's a saying that goes. "I can resist anything except temptation!"

To think that some people ran around galavanting during covid-19 and holiday times. Is another story. But not unfathomable. A word had been started by now. From frontline workers who were overwhelmed. "Super-spreaders." Because this is exactly what was happening.

Now if you were like me. Then maybe you thought. That the last days could be near. Then I can understand your logic and rebellious bucket list mentality! There's a difference between smart and stupid. To travel during those times was totally absurd! And actually outright disrespectful. Especially when trying to set unachievable standards or goals.

The requirement of maintaining stay-at-home protocol from officials wasn't a tall task at all. In the grand scheme of things. If you look at the fact that people were traveling just because they could. It shows a level of entitlement.

I mean never had people felt so privileged to travel. But maybe at the expense of others made it more disheartening. Of course sickening. All while a certain medical procedure was gaining steam like a locomotive. The vaccinations were rumored to be effective.

#15
VACCINATIONS

On December 2, 2020. A European country became the first to authorize a coronavirus (covid-19)) vaccination. That was a historic day. In terms of being a worldwide monumental milestone. It was groundbreaking! The country where it just happened to be approved was hit hard. The death toll was astonishing! As much debilitating and heartbreaking. People fell on hard times. We just needed our country to follow suit.

In the matter of about a week. Advances were made in the lovely home of the brave. A medical company was granted authorized emergency use on December 10, 2020.

With the news grew groans. Especially since. The outlets had let the cat out of the bag on mass vaccinations! See at the time precisely. I didn't see the exact logic. That this new drug would conquer coronavirus.

Like who said so? I was opposed to the idea and thought of taking some new medicine. But empathically cared enough to support it. Accordingly to the elderly with underlining issues.

The mistreatment of the elderly was simply despicable. I mean this was somebody's Grandma, Grandpa, Uncle, Aunt, and so on. I couldn't believe it! Even if I thought my mind was playing tricks on me!

Those images still haunt me. But the medical advancements were more. Then just an expedited process! If life has shown us anything. It's you can't cut corners with extremely high rates of speed. And not expect a crash!

The vaccantions for coronavirus aka covid-19 were needed. To not only curve the deadly virus. But too show the public the officials respected the older generations. That life mattered no matter your age!

Knowing that in the 21st century. There could have been a plague? Maybe it could've helped us better prepare for the deadly virus. But that's a hypothetical! Because just as we were preparing for the mass distribution of the medicine.

There came all types of scenarios. From the dual administered two-shot cocktail. To a single shot booster. And maybe a three-shot trial run. That was enough to have me leary of this new medicine. This vaccination! And I wasn't the only skeptical one.

From the beginning of the talk about vaccinations. I was really interested in hearing every bit of information. I could get. The times called for it! My logic was there. I did everything as if my life depended on it.

I researched everything I could from the normal, not computer literate perspective. As I did during time. I watched a lot of early morning media outlets. Trying to maintain a disciplined approach to life. I didn't trust something!

Just like everybody else. I felt you can't just emergency authorize something. Especially something new. I can remember a lot of people having a theory of being test dummies and guinea pigs. Sad measure.

See coronavirus had a catatrophic effect. People were dying and scared. The last thing they wanted to do was. Put some new medicine in their bodies. That they knew nothing about! That could possibly kill and have life-long side effects.

During the highest times of hospitalizations since the pandemic hit. The advancements in medical procedures and technology were a necessarily rushed effort. As much as it was deemed as. "The weapon that wins the covid war!" We have to give science credit.

The rate of death from coronavirus was depressing! Especially for the elderly with underlining issues. So putting them a high priority was a major step in the right direction. Even though the mistreatment of senior citizens was seriously neglected by some state officials. Everything would eventually come to light.

So with nursing homes, targeted as a high priority! Because of risk and exposure due to coronavirus aka covid-19. Also the death rate! The trickle-down effect was in place. The nursing home residents and frontline workers would be the first to receive vaccinations.

My specific area was to receive 170,000 vaccines. That was to be maintained at a certain temperature of minus 70 degrees celsus. The vaccinations would be needed to be stored and mass-distributed at an exact temperature.

Special freezers were brought in and dry ice to help keep the temperatures of vaccines maintained. We faced another challenge with not only the leeriness of people. But undisciplined citizens and unnecessary travel.

The first to be administered a vaccination shot to combat coronavirus was a 90-year-old woman overseas. It was uplifting to see targeting the older and more susceptible to coronavirus get first shots.

Also protecting the very people who risked exposure. Put their lives on the line! Each and every second, minute, and hour. It felt like we were taking steps in the right direction toward moving forward. And maybe to having a coronavirus-free world.

See as predicted by experts and doctors. We were moving into unprecedented times of coronavirus aka covid-19 infections and hospitalizations. With the vaccinations emergency approval came another hurdle.

Not only were the months ahead deemed the worst and darkest. If that wasn't a scare factor to get people to try a drug. I don't know what is! The spike remained inevitable. As people traveled like there wasn't anything wrong. Our selfish act of deviancy affected the mass distribution of vaccinations and maintenance of coronavirus.

#16
HERD IMMUNITY

While people were galavanting like it was the end of the world. Double-checking off Miami. Those unnecessary trips almost slowed down the entire process of distribution. As I watched more informative shows on vaccinations every day. I started to be intrigued based on a social media live.

The fellow was speaking about how the vaccine was being administered. Who? When? and What? As he spoke I listened to close tuning in my spidey senses.

The young man was articulate. Also knew a lot of what I was into at the time. Information! As he spoke more from a vivid point of how to maneuver around during covid. He stressed the point.

That as much as it seemed like the older generations and frontline workers, were to be prioritized. That wasn't truly the issue. It was money! And the wealthy were lining up fast.

See what he was speaking was right. There would be no doubt that the wealthy were going to get their first dibs. I believed him. Next, he said something that almost through me in a time warp.

His exact words were "Herd immunity!" Hearing it then. I can say now I almost freaked out. I remember thinking about some mad cow disease in humans. It's no doubt, I was confused!

The thought of a herd as people. I didn't get it! But the immunity part. I totally understood. Especially in terms. Of the scientific fact that as much as studies showed that Blacks, Latinos, and the poor are more susceptible to coronavirus. Blacks have a 2 to 1 death rate.

The more I listened to that live. For at least an hour and a half! It was obvious, that his insight was right! Coronavirus had trademark transmissions in communities of color. And death was right around the corner.

To think that the authorization of emergency use of vaccinations to combat coronavirus was a scare tactic. Wasn't beyond the unimaginable creative mind. But from a logical standpoint. Some of the things just didn't add up!

Especially when I looked into everything! Herd immunity's most basic meaning is resistance to the spread of an infectious disease within a population. That is based on pre-existing immunity of a high proportion of individuals! As a result of previous infection or vaccinations.

Simple in plain. I was more nervous about the thought of the side effects of coronavirus vaccinations. Then the number game and percentage. Our leaders were starting to endorse. The country would promote at an exceedingly fast rate the shot. Trying to achieve a number of 75% to 85% percent of citizens vaccinated.

See with that number being set. I can honestly say. It felt as if we were finally moving into numerological historical times. That a number had to be set. There was a slim glimmer of hope. That coronavirus aka covid-19. Could and maybe would be eradicated from human being civilization.

The more I felt leary of the vaccinations. As much as I journaled every day, morning, noon, and night. I became more informed on the side effects of coronavirus. As people were being administered vaccination shots every day now. With that came the scientific-fact-based information experimentation. A lot of people reported feeling yucky!

Which was expected like in every other shot given. But when I heard the news of a nurse fainting after getting shot. I was convinced. I wasn't getting it!!!

Just like most Americans. At this exact time in history. I was scared, I was nervous. I mean there is something about it. The fear of the unknown. I personally understood and didn't trust. Putting a new medicine in my body! I knew it could have side effects. I could care less about herd immunity or Quality of life.

#16 Deemed dark time/Changing of guard

This time in my life was easily the hardest of any time. I mean coming home from prison. It wasn't at all about some perfect life. I can remember going to that job interview. For a job as they so-called an essential worker. More like entitlement worker! Like honestly my interviewer had a patch over his eye. Which wasn't really the problem. But maybe he was blind to something.

To me, there was something about being gainfully employed. That motivated me each and every day. When I wasn't motivated. I know I had outstanding attendance. I had a certain quality of joy.

I mean pre-covid. I did enjoy the commute and working at the store. I think that was my genuine side showing unconditional love from the average guy. Also feeling like a productive member of society.

I mean then I needed the job. I was making less than a minimum wage before my job in retail. My hours didn't add up to my previous lifestyle.

So I went to a job that might have been a shortstop. But I never noticed how the sport baseball. Could've played a part in my American history.

I remember going away and saying. I had three baseball seasons. But that was in terms of past time. Coming home and working at retail store. Maybe wasn't right for me at all!

But as we dwelled on a historic time when the average American was in the hardest or harshest time of times. I was pressed to go back to work.

See at the time. As unemployment scams were at an all-time high. I had walked away from the retail job. As much as tried to appeal an unemployment decision. I got nothing.

So as time moved forward to be efficient, effective, and last but not least responsible. I had to go back to work. I only had one stipulation. I wasn't working with any customers.

Overtime! This was not an easy task. I mean at the darkest of times of hospitalizations for coronavirus and death. I wasn't working. I wasn't being self-sufficient. I know having a moral principle was right. But maybe not feasible. I needed a new normal or a Quality of life. I never knew of existed?

#17
LOOKING FOR WORK

I remember filling out the first dozens of applications. Then what felt like hundreds. As more time passed. We remained in a dark time! I was scared. But somewhat fearless! To a lot that. I knew nothing about it.

I guess I was stepping out on faith. I still journaled about coronavirus daily. The stuff I was hearing about from side effects. Wasn't of the norm. So I tried to keep up.

A quality time of life and a herd immunity didn't add up. Especially to the simple bills I had. So how did that figure into most Americans' lives? At the time I was down and out bad like a Kayne West song!

So looking forward to news outlets talking about a new normal. Also some relief packages. The timing was off. The amounts were a little short. But I was very appreciative of everything!

In a matter of time. As watched intently on new ways the world was changing. It wasn't just the beginning about finding some newfound lifestyle. I mean I was literally still in the trenches.

As I watched everybody go up. I questioned myself. The system. I mean at times. I felt the system didn't protect the hard-working. Boy was I right.

I can remember the day like it was yesterday. The date now was about March of 2021. Stimulus packages were going out. But since I wasn't a direct deposit recipient. It took a little longer for my payment.

I had been overwhelmed. Even heard family members say I was a burden. My mental health was a wreck. It's like I said before it's hard for a person to rationalize when they fucked up.

Things for me somehow. Someway were changing. Even though to the eye. I was broken. Physically, mentally, and last but not least financially.

At this time for me. It honestly might have been the hardest time of my life. Something had to change. My mentality was something had to break!

I kept looking for jobs and around April. I received my relief package. I thought I was in for a break. Because I knew I was willing to go back to work. Just not work with people. I mean customers.

#18
JOURNALING

Journaling by now had become a hobby. I woke to the news and looked at any headline with amazement. There was something about the information marketing field. I knew nothing about it.

Soon as I researched everything under sun and moon. On coronavirus, vaccinations, and its side effects. I not only became amazed. But empathetic, convalescent, and more passionate.

One morning as I woke up. I usually collected info. But since I did this daily. Now I just listened. It wasn't anything about anything in particular. But maybe a mental drain!

I really needed something to help my sufficiency level. That day as I moved around oblivious to what was about to happen. I took the time to notice. I was falling in love with writing.

"Writing didn't pay bills!" My people had just told me that! But it somehow created a space in my heart, mind, body, and soul! That I never had.

I was now eagerly and silently anticipating something great. I was passionate about it. I took the time for it. But I didn't appreciate it. As one of the strongest forms of communication!

Then I mean was told I wrote some nice letters. It's different though when you are gathering information! On another level! That's promoted to the masses about their health, safety, and determent too infectious diseases! Also, it's medicine! A vaccine.

I don't think I noticed the full impact of coronavirus on my people or me. Until I had a sort of isolation during the deemed dark time. See myself I knew the impact. That one bad decision in indecision about the health of others! Could be drastic to somebody else! Especially family!

As much as I was opposed to the vaccine. I wasn't at all opinionated. When it came to the older generation with underlining health issues. If u were.

In our world, at the time you were termed a covid-idiot. I mean people were really dying. What made it worse was some people thought they had the right to question if somebody got it!

This was pure comedy because some were anti-vaccine like me. They just didn't have the know that or wherewithal to go or not go. Let alone valuable information! This created debauchery to herd immunity.

The government was trying to create a vaccinated shield against coronavirus and combat it! I think it was for the quality of life for people! And the new normal. But as time went by and more people got vaccinated. Especially family! I felt a changing of the guard.

A lot of this gave to optimism for better days to come. Where we were coronavirus free. Or it was obsolete. Happiness for me to accomplish the impossible. People like me look for opportunities and take them seriously.

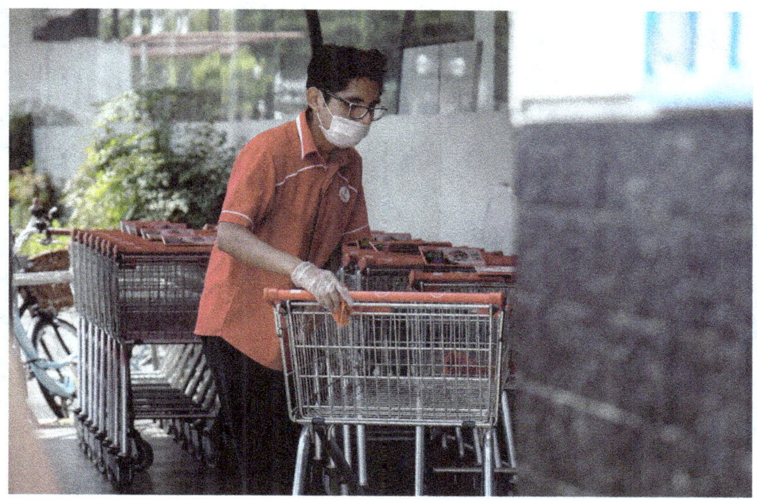

So one day as I heard the news on my local news channel. I had heard so much flooded coronavirus material. It didn't ring in my ears that particular day. Yea new normal this. New normal that!

Something was about to happen though. There as I listened getting ready for my day! I heard a news lady's voice sound so elegant. She spoke of a entrpeneurship program. That if completed would help you get a 5,000.00 dollar grant for small business. I immediately jotted the information down. "Westchester Launch 1000!"

Later that day. I used my mobile device to search " Westchester Launch 1000". What I saw possessed. The best view in town! So that itself was very intriguing.

I filled out all the info. Applying for this program made me feel. An infinite potential. Honestly, that before covid never would have been found.

In terms of the quality of life. That is what doctors, state officials, and world leaders were telling or informing us about. It sounded really good! About how the coronavirus vaccinations were going to end the covid war. We just needed a lot of people to get vaccinated to create this herd immunity!

They promoted vaccinations from every angle possible. They didn't miss one public service announcement for this or that! Even the debriefing was very different.

While they looked like heroes. So much was brewing inside. I see why I questioned everything and everybody on the outside! Because most have an ulterior motive. Especially higher-ups!

This was a tumultuous time for most! I mean not only were you afraid of the thought of coronavirus and death. But also thought of vaccination was horrifying to some like me. Looking back you had a double standard going!

Some wanted to get vaccinated. But feared backlash from family members at local functions. It took a strong personality who stood up to confrontation! On their health, strict morals, principles, and beliefs. Not just travel.

To think some were getting vaccinated to travel was another. Here we go again moment. Like if your life depended on it. People were ready to check off the bucket list!

All while some didn't have jobs. Like myself. Which helped us see the selfish arrogant opinionated side of people!

When my family got vaccinated. I totally understood. As much as I wanted to complain. About what, I didn't know about the vaccine? I fully supported them and it! The hot topic had crossed our dinner table.

I can remember as the weather got better and sweatier. I received an email from a contract management company named Entrepreneur Ready! The name had a ring to it.

"Oh, this from Westchester launch 1000." I read information more as I applied for a free computer. Which was needed to complete the program. And since I didn't have one the county was donating one for me.

A great way to get to the resources. See then I didn't understand computers. Actually, I didn't even see any problem! Then with not having one. But since I didn't have one. I thought I could use one. When I was emailed back with instructions on when, where, and time to pick up the computer. I felt a newfound sense

#20
PERFECT TIMING

Sometimes things just happen at the right time. I was calling around after getting news from Entrepreneur Ready. When I started doing follow-ups for applications. I had filled out in the area. There had to be a certain aura over me! Because here is where the story gets good or interesting.

My first follow-up call was with a local clothing drive. I had been calling that company for about a month. With no luck! That day though I spoke with somebody in position. Who just happened to take notice of my initiative.

About a day later. I received a call from the clothing drive. Telling me to come in for an interview. I was shocked! It was the same day. I was to pick up the computer from the entrepreneurship program. There felt like a good chance. I was going to soon be gainfully employed again. My destiny and fate would soon play out.

The exact date was June 4, 2021. I went to the county office to pick up a loaner computer. As the program wasn't accessible for mobile devices or smartphones at the time. The elegance of the office was appealing. I felt I was in the right place! I saw some county big wigs. It felt like something about ideas was going on. The woman who gave me the computer was very detailed oriented!

After our introduction. When she told me. That, if I completed the program. I could keep the computer. I was appalled. I didn't know. That at the time, would be the best thing happening in my life! I signed for the computer. We exchanged best wishes and farewells!

To think as I walked off. That by having a computer in one of those tote bags. I felt a different aura about life is an understatement. My walk was with confidence. As I made my way to the clothing drive. There was no doubt I felt I was getting a job. I just worried about vaccine protocol!

See some jobs weren't hiring without vaccination. I prayed on it a little bit. But when I arrived and met the manager. I felt a cool homeboy-type swag.

The manager showed me around. And soon was telling me everything. When he offered me the job! I was stunned. I felt somebody was giving me another opportunity. And I wouldn't let them down!

#21
THE COMPANY

For the clothing drive, you didn't have to be vaccinated. I went into that job and started working a 2 to 10 shift. Agreeing to work 6 days a week. I had just been out of work for 8 months. So it felt like I was behind the 8-ball. I was to start the very next day!

Looking back. I went into that job. With great intentions. But definitely with blinders on My job was as a material handler. I was to unload and load donated clothes on and off company trucks.

What I thought I liked about this job. It was in a very interesting area. One I frequented. Also had childhood friends. So the motivation was there!

It only took a little bit of time. Actually about a week. I saw progress in myself! A lot of questioning or worry about coronavirus? Seemed like they weren't there anymore. I worked hard and stayed focused! Locking in!

When that first check came. I was jubilant! I had just made double the money in a week. Then I made, at the grocery store. This also was a two-week pay system. That check began to give me the basis of reality. That some jobs don't give a fuck about you.

There's nothing wrong with working hard for a company. I was destined by that first check. I tried to make those numbers every pay period. I was working like 60 to 70 hours a week. Really dedicated to my position and making sure my work was done efficiently.

To say, I went into that job a little naive. Is the truth! Looking back honestly, I'm like every human. As much as I wasn't dealing with customers directly. I only saw the opportunity. I never could imagine the inner workings. Of a business so fast.

The "Company" supposedly followed covid-19 protocol. Workers were to wear masks. But with conditions of sweltering heat with no air conditioning. It made the job almost unbearable especially while wearing a mask. I noticed something about this company! I was working for was compromising my breathing.

Now there's nothing wrong with a compromise. As long as two sides are mutually agreed upon. If you remember most of this is about the ramifications of coronavirus and its deaths. Also possible side effects of the vaccinations. I had no problem working hard! I just wasn't going to die for it!

Life is precious and should be treated accordingly. Again the way, I was working at this company was beyond tremendous. To a point one day. I unloaded 4,000 pounds of donated clothes off a truck and baled 2,000 pounds. Made me understand! I was born in America song! "Made in America"

The time at that time wasn't the best. But this company. Since I had been out of work minus covid mandates made me work my ass off. I mean I really worked hard. I didn't know exactly, if it was an opportunity. Until one day I took my computer to work.

If u told me something about coronavirus changing the world? I can honestly say. I would've looked at you weird! But as time sped up. The estimation of herd immunity couldn't have been more off. That is in a matter of months of consistent work! The company told me to lag off hours.

I sort of couldn't believe it. But I accepted everything. Until I was working a complete shift by myself. It was like everything, I had learned was changing. I think of my infinite potential and possibilities. Reverted right there. In those moments. Inside an empty truck. Where and when no one else showed up.

Soon covid-19 vaccinations were pushing full-throttle. Rumors began of the company having a mandate for workers. I began to question and doubt myself all over again. I mean this job. This company! That was giving me an estimated value of great pay for a prisoner coming home. Couldn't have helped me notice something?

There's a saying. "You never get paid what you worth, but what you negotiate!" I had no clue I had just coerced myself. Until a life-changing compromise. The company would soon place a vaccination order over all employees.

I can remember co-workers and friends asking me. "If I was getting it?" I had no direct answers. My self-sufficiency and sustainability had been put into question. I had nothing. The company had me by the balls.

The one thing I did have? What I never took into account was this program from Westchester Launch 1000 and Entrepreneur Ready. I went on a few zoom calls. But my vision was still blurry!

The things I worked on while working. For this company was instrumental in my life! My life had a lot of flaws. As much, as I will admit I enjoyed hearing entrepreneurship talks. I had some serious interpersonal skills. I had to work on and learn to network.

I started to grasp things better. See a clearer vision. I remember one day at work seeing this amazingly beautiful woman with a vibrant soul! We spoke. I just would never know. How ironic and iconic that meeting was.

Working for companies will have you comprise. Almost all your ethics, principles, and moral codes. See I had a vision, but not really at the perseverance level I needed. My balance system was still off. Missing a few more things?

"The Entrepreneur Ready program was a blessing in disguise!" I remember thinking? Like how else do I get passive income, teach, speak, and help others? On all the platforms I dreamed of.

But with resistance from the public to get vaccinated. The higher-ups started to have jobs that gave pay incentives for getting vaccinated. This was now the new rumor at "The company."

One difference between a rumor is some have the truth. As I worked my ass off. I challenged myself to complete the entrepreneurship-ready program. I felt they were was a lot of infinite potential in it for me!

Just like life is one day as I went to work. I was informed by the supervisor of a date to be vaccinated. I knew my life was going to change.

I knew I had just found some consistency. It also meant something to do things. Effectively and efficiently! I had no care for herd immunity or quality of life. All I cared about was never going back to life! Where I wasn't self-sufficient.

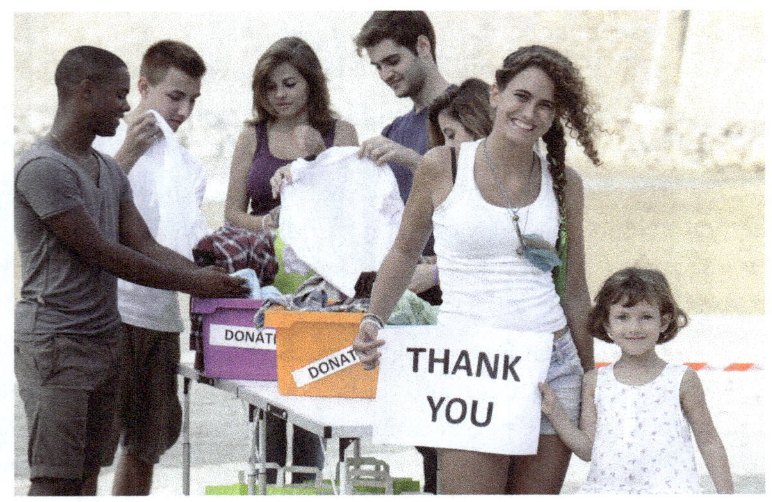

So I went and planned to get vaccinated. While a lot will question. How? Why? What? One thing that life shows you is? The opinionated side of someone else!

#23 VACCINATED/ LETTER OF GULIT

Who psychologically will make it like you did something wrong. When it's something wrong with those over-critical pessimistic narcissists' point-of-views. I mean people were just dying. If there are two things coronavirus or covid-19 had showed us. It was death and taxes was real!

I went and got vaccinated around my birthday Sept 4th. It was a day. I had to work. So I called myself. With the workaholic mentality. After getting a shot and vac card!

Going to work. I can remember questioning myself. Like when I signed a letter of guilt. Those moments made me second-guess myself completely.

I remember walking that day a little wobbly. I started my shift. Maybe worked an hour. Then felt nausea! The excruciating heat. On and off a truck. In a sweltering hot warehouse combined together with. What else the vaccine had its side effects on me. I left work for that day!

Resting up and drinking a lot of water and vitamin c. I emerged later the next day a new man. I felt my work plan and life was headed for good fortunes. I continued to work my ass off. Head down, locked in doing the work! There was a lot of growth those days.

With my growth, I started to notice everything. The company was now showing signs of dysfunction and incompetence in management. So much my name came up. Because of tremendous work ethic. For managerial position. While management chooses to go in another direction.

I worked the entrepreneur program. Phase after phase. I learned about business planning, target market, and scientific facts! Recipes, secret sauce, and sweet spots. I took to the education. Over video confernces! One thing covid had just validated in me was. I wasn't going to let somebody else out research me.

Information for me was more vital and valuable than ever. See I didn't run and get shot. But what I did was give myself the best shot to win. Oh I have to say that again. "Best shot to win."

There's something about self-sufficiency. That gave me the big game shot-taker mentality. From Jordan to Kobe to Bird to Magic. You knew who was going to get shot and there was nothing. U could do to them stop them!

Herd immunity was the defense. Quality of life was the offense. So you know what they say? "Better offense beats better defense!' They were both at hand.

And too think, I wasn't even ambidextrous! I don't know why? But I was more confident than usual. So confident one day? I went to work. I was told to not punch in.

I thought aw shit! What the fuck! I was directed to the front office. Then given a letter informing me of the company's downsizing. Long story short! I had just been laid off. I couldn't believe it. But I thanked them anyway for the opportunity.

#24
LAIDOFF/ APPLYING PRESSURE

I remember first being upset about getting vaccinated. Then the company. Laying me off! But I applied for unemployment. Then really locked into Entrepreneur Ready. I had only two phases left.

Looking back. Trying to complete that program and work 60 to 70 hours. Was obtainable. Probably a little outlandish. Especially overwhelming on the mind, body, and soul!

Not only was the psychological thought of covid. A difference-maker for me. I wanted to dream of financial freedom. Writing literacy programs! My vision was different. I'm forever thankful for the coronavirus because it taught me not only death. But to work from home was possible.

I always dreamed of writing a book. That I felt was influential enough. That I just had to get it published. Now to be able to. Also teach these moments are the joys of life. I mean the stuff some persevere a lifetime of hurt, pain, and loss!

Then overcome all thw negativity and defeat! Was a victory itself. but im not into moral victories! For me, it's a satisfaction to see others have the benefit of joy, health, wealth, and wellness. It's a game-changer for me.

If we had a chance to go back? And inexperience the whole covid-19 thing over! I'm pretty sure, we all would have done it over. Better prepared! I mean showing less resistance to the innovative advanced medical procedures.

That did prove effective and efficient! While creating herd immunity. Which was celebrated across the country by the government!

I don't think you had to tell me. About misinformation and miscalculations on coronavirus deaths. Because so many real-life scenarios existed. But so much was going on on the medical front. That something was going on in all forms of government.

From Federal or state. To think the covid epidemic was part of any corruption. Is beyond plausible. From the President to the Governor of one of the world's largest cities. We fell on infamous historical times! Some were neglected. Some had no lack of respect and called it patriotism! But one thing remained death.

Some of us emerged from covid-19! Like me motivated. Informed and detailed oriented. Things I never was because of never really experiencing sacrifice, isolation, dedication, and finally. Thinking outside the box. Creatively. Defining my intellectual property.

Because finally, my decision for becoming a small business would become a reality! An achieved lifetime goal. Skillset Writers! Dedicated to culture! By helping everyday people write books based on real authentic relatable stories based on empathetic convalescent healing. The end !!!!!

Reid Skillset